KETO DIET RECIPES

THE MOST DELICIOUS MEAT AND VEGETABLE RECIPES TO LOSE WEIGHT AND BE MORE ENERGETIC

DONALD FRIEDMAN

Table of Contents

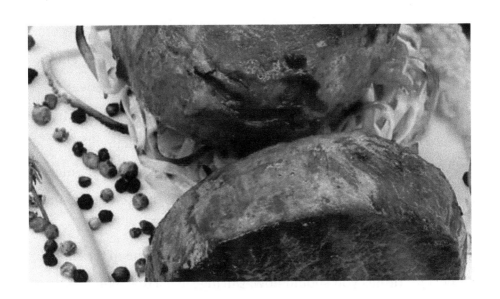

Introduction

Do you want to make a change in your life? Do you want to become a healthier person who can enjoy a new and improved life? Then, you are definitely in the right place. You are about to discover a wonderful and very healthy diet that has changed millions of lives. We are talking about the Ketogenic diet, a lifestyle that will mesmerize you and that will make you a new person in no time. So, let's sit back, relax and find out more about the Ketogenic diet.

A keto diet is a low carb one. This is the first and one of the most important things you should now. During such a diet, your body makes ketones in your liver and these are used as energy.
Your body will produce less insulin and glucose and a state of ketosis is induced.
Ketosis is a natural process that appears when our food intake is lower than usual. The body will soon adapt to this state and therefore you will be able to lose weight in no time but you will also become healthier and your physical and mental performances will improve.
Your blood sugar levels will improve and you won't be predisposed to diabetes.

Also, epilepsy and heart diseases can be prevented if you are on a Ketogenic diet.

Your cholesterol will improve and you will feel amazing in no time. How does that sound?

A Ketogenic diet is simple and easy to follow as long as you follow some simple rules. You don't need to make huge changes but there are some things you should know.

So, here goes!

If you are on a Ketogenic diet you can't eat:

- Grains like corn, cereals, rice, etc
- Fruits like bananas
- Sugar
- Dry beans
- Honey
- Potatoes
- Yams

If you are on a Ketogenic diet you can eat:

- Greens like spinach, green beans, kale, bok choy, etc
- Meat like poultry, fish, pork, lamb, beef, etc
- Eggs
- Above ground veggies like cauliflower or broccoli, napa cabbage or regular cabbage
- Nuts and seeds
- Cheese
- Ghee or butter
- Avocados and all kind of berries
- Sweeteners like erythritol, splenda, stevia and others that contain only a few carbs
- Coconut oil
- Avocado oil
- Olive oil

The list of foods you are allowed to eat during a keto diet is permissive and rich as you can see for yourself.

So, we think it should be pretty easy for you to start such a diet.

If you've made this choice already, then, it's time you checked our amazing keto recipe collection.

You will discover 50 of the best Ketogenic Meat and Vegetable recipes in the world and you will soon be able to make each and every one of these recipes.

Now let's start our magical culinary journey!
Ketogenic lifestyle...here we come!
Enjoy!

Ketogenic Meat Recipes

Cuban Beef Stew

A Cuban keto stew can make your day a lot better!

Preparation time: 10 minutes

Cooking time: 6 hours

Servings: 8

Ingredients:

- 2 yellow onions, chopped
- 2 tablespoons avocado oil
- 2 pounds beef roast, cubed
- 2 green bell peppers, chopped
- 1 habanero pepper, chopped
- 4 jalapenos, chopped
- 14 ounces canned tomatoes, chopped
- 2 tablespoons cilantro, chopped
- 6 garlic cloves, minced
- ½ cup water
- Salt and black pepper to the taste
- 1 and ½ teaspoons cumin, ground
- 4 teaspoons bouillon granules
- ½ cup black olives, pitted and chopped
- 1 teaspoon oregano, dried

Directions:

1. Heat up a pan with the oil over medium high heat, add beef, brown it on all sides and transfer to a slow cooker.
2. Add green bell peppers, onions, jalapenos, habanero pepper, tomatoes, garlic, water, bouillon, cilantro, oregano, cumin, salt and pepper and stir.
3. Cover slow cooker and cook on Low for 6 hours.
4. Add olives, stir, divide into bowls and serve.

Enjoy!

Nutrition: calories 305, fat 14, fiber 4, carbs 8, protein 25

Ham Stew

It's perfect for dinner tonight!

Preparation time: 10 minutes

Cooking time: 4 hours

Servings: 6

Ingredients:

- 8 ounces cheddar cheese, grated
- 14 ounces chicken stock
- ½ teaspoon garlic powder
- ½ teaspoon onion powder
- Salt and black pepper to the taste
- 4 garlic cloves, minced
- ¼ cup heavy cream
- 3 cups ham, chopped
- 16 ounces cauliflower florets

Directions:

1. In your Crockpot, mix ham with stock, cheese, cauliflower, garlic powder, onion powder, salt, pepper, garlic and heavy cream, stir, cover and cook on High for 4 hours.

2. Stir, divide into bowls and serve.

Enjoy!

Nutrition: calories 320, fat 20, fiber 3, carbs 6, protein 23

Delicious Veal Stew

No matter how busy you are, you can make the time to prepare this keto dish!

Preparation time: 10 minutes

Cooking time: 2 hours and 10 minutes

Servings: 12

Ingredients:

- 2 tablespoons avocado oil
- 3 pounds veal, cubed
- 1 yellow onion, chopped
- 1 small garlic clove, minced
- Salt and black pepper to the taste
- 1 cup water
- 1 and ½ cups marsala wine
- 10 ounces canned tomato paste
- 1 carrot, chopped
- 7 ounces mushrooms, chopped
- 3 egg yolks
- ½ cup heavy cream
- 2 teaspoons oregano, dried

Directions:

1. Heat up a pot with the oil over medium high heat, add veal, stir and brown it for a few minutes.
2. Add garlic and onion, stir and cook for 2-3 minutes more.
3. Add wine, water, oregano, tomato paste, mushrooms, carrots, salt and pepper, stir, bring to a boil, cover, reduce heat to low and cook for 1 hour and 45 minutes.
4. In a bowl, mix cream with egg yolks and whisk well.
5. Pour this into the pot, stir, cook for 15 minutes more, add more salt and pepper if needed, divide into bowls and serve.

Enjoy!

Nutrition: calories 254, fat 15, fiber 1, carbs 3, protein 23

Veal And Tomatoes Dish

Make a special dinner for your loved ones! Try this keto recipe!

Preparation time: 10 minutes

Cooking time: 40 minutes

Servings: 4

Ingredients:

- 4 medium veal leg steaks
- A drizzle of avocado oil
- 2 garlic cloves, minced
- 1 red onion, chopped
- Salt and black pepper to the taste
- 2 teaspoons sage, chopped
- 15 ounces canned tomatoes, chopped
- 2 tablespoons parsley, chopped
- 1 ounce bocconcini, sliced
- Green beans, steamed for serving

Directions:

1. Heat up a pan with the oil over medium high heat, add veal, cook for 2 minutes on each side and transfer to a baking dish.

17

2. Return pan to heat, add onion, stir and cook for 4 minutes.

3. Add sage and garlic, stir and cook for 1 minute.

4. Add tomatoes, stir, bring to a boil and cook for 10 minutes.

5. Pour this over veal, add bocconcini and parsley, introduce in the oven at 350 degrees G and bake for 20 minutes.

6. Divide between plates and serve with steamed green beans on the side.

Enjoy!

Nutrition: calories 276, fat 6, fiber 4, carbs 5, protein 36

Veal Parmesan

It's a very popular keto dish and you should learn how to make it!

Preparation time: 10 minutes

Cooking time: 1 hour and 10 minutes

Servings: 6

Ingredients:

- 8 veal cutlets
- 2/3 cup parmesan, grated
- 8 provolone cheese slices
- Salt and black pepper to the taste
- 5 cups tomato sauce
- A pinch of garlic salt
- Cooking spray
- 2 tablespoons ghee
- 2 tablespoons coconut oil, melted
- 1 teaspoon Italian seasoning

Directions:

1. Season veal cutlets with salt, pepper and garlic salt,

2. Heat up a pan with the ghee and the oil over medium high heat, add veal and cook until they brown on all sides.
3. Spread half of the tomato sauce on the bottom of a baking dish which you've greased with some cooking spray.
4. Add veal cutlets, then sprinkle Italian seasoning and spread the rest of the sauce.
5. Cover dish, introduce in the oven at 350 degrees F and bake for 40 minutes.
6. Uncover dish, spread provolone cheese and sprinkle parmesan, introduce in the oven again and bake for 15 minutes more.
7. Divide between plates and serve.

Enjoy!

Nutrition: calories 362, fat 21, fiber 2, carbs 6, protein 26

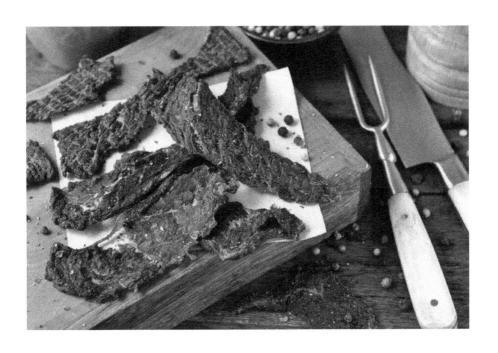

Veal Piccata

Make this for your loved one tonight!

Preparation time: 10 minutes

Cooking time: 15 minutes

Servings: 2

Ingredients:

- 2 tablespoons ghee
- ¼ cup white wine
- ¼ cup chicken stock
- 1 and ½ tablespoons capers
- 1 garlic clove, minced
- 8 ounces veal scallops
- Salt and black pepper to the taste

Directions:

1. Heat up a pan with half of the butter over medium high heat, add veal cutlets, season with salt and pepper, cook for 1 minute on each side and transfer to a plate.
2. Heat up the pan again over medium heat, add garlic, stir and cook for 1 minute.
3. Add wine, stir and simmer for 2 minutes.

4. Add stock, capers, salt, pepper, the rest of the ghee and return veal to pan.
5. Stir everything, cover pan and cook piccata on medium low heat until veal is tender.

Enjoy!

Nutrition: calories 204, fat 12, fiber 1, carbs 5, protein 10

Delicious Roasted Sausage

It's very easy to make at home tonight!

Preparation time: 10 minutes

Cooking time: 1 hour

Servings: 6

Ingredients:

- 3 red bell peppers, chopped
- 2 pounds Italian pork sausage, sliced
- Salt and black pepper to the taste
- 2 pounds Portobello mushrooms, sliced
- 2 sweet onions, chopped
- 1 tablespoon swerve
- A drizzle of olive oil

Directions:

1. In a baking dish, mix sausage slices with oil, salt, pepper, bell pepper, mushrooms, onion and swerve.
2. Toss to coat, introduce in the oven at 300 degrees F and bake for 1 hour.
3. Divide between plates and serve hot.

Enjoy!

Nutrition: calories 130, fat 12, fiber 1, carbs 3, protein 9

Baked Sausage And Kale

This keto dish will be ready in 20 minutes!

Preparation time: 5 minutes

Cooking time: 30 minutes

Servings: 4

Ingredients:

- 1 cup yellow onion, chopped
- 1 and ½ pound Italian pork sausage, sliced
- ½ cup red bell pepper, chopped
- Salt and black pepper to the taste
- 5 pounds kale, chopped
- 1 teaspoon garlic, minced
- ¼ cup red hot chili pepper, chopped
- 1 cup water

Directions:

1. Heat up a pan over medium high heat, add sausage, stir, reduce heat to medium and cook for 10 minutes.
2. Add onions, stir and cook for 3-4 minutes more.
3. Add bell pepper and garlic, stir and cook for 1 minute.

4. Add kale, chili pepper, salt, pepper and water, stir and cook for 10 minutes more.

5. Divide between plates and serve.

Enjoy!

Nutrition: calories 150, fat 4, fiber 1, carbs 2, protein 12

Sausage With Tomatoes And Cheese

It's a surprising and very tasty combination!

Preparation time: 10 minutes

Cooking time: 30 minutes

Servings: 4

Ingredients:

- 2 ounces coconut oil, melted
- 2 pounds Italian pork sausage, chopped
- 1 onion, sliced
- 4 sun-dried tomatoes, thinly sliced
- Salt and black pepper to the taste
- ½ pound gouda cheese, grated
- 3 yellow bell peppers, chopped
- 3 orange bell peppers, chopped
- A pinch of red pepper flakes
- A handful parsley, thinly sliced

Directions:

1. Heat up a pan with the oil over medium high heat, add sausage slices, stir, cook for 3 minutes on each side, transfer to a plate and leave aside for now.

28

2. Heat up the pan again over medium heat, add onion, yellow and orange bell peppers and tomatoes, stir and cook for 5 minutes.
3. Add pepper flakes, salt and pepper, stir well, cook for 1 minute and take off heat.
4. Arrange sausage slices into a baking dish, add bell peppers mix on top, add parsley and gouda as well, introduce in the oven at 350 degrees F and bake for 15 minutes.
5. Divide between plates and serve hot.

Enjoy!

Nutrition: calories 200, fat 5, fiber 3, carbs 6, protein 14

Delicious Sausage Salad

Check this out! It's very tasty!

Preparation time: 10 minutes

Cooking time: 7 minutes

Servings: 4

Ingredients:

- 8 pork sausage links, sliced
- 1 pound mixed cherry tomatoes, cut in halves
- 4 cups baby spinach
- 1 tablespoon avocado oil
- 1 pound mozzarella cheese, cubed
- 2 tablespoons lemon juice
- 2/3 cup basil pesto
- Salt and black pepper to the taste

Directions:

1. Heat up a pan with the oil over medium high heat, add sausage slices, stir and cook them for 4 minutes on each side.

2. Meanwhile, in a salad bowl, mix spinach with mozzarella, tomatoes, salt, pepper, lemon juice and pesto and toss to coat.

3. Add sausage pieces, toss again and serve.

Enjoy!

Nutrition: calories 250, fat 12, fiber 3, carbs 8, protein 18

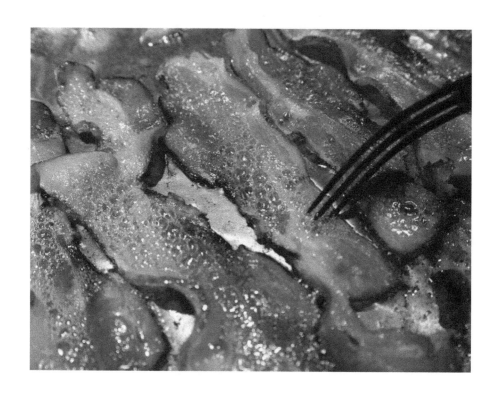

Delicious Sausage And Peppers Soup

This keto soup will hypnotize everyone!

Preparation time: 10 minutes

Cooking time: 1 hour and 10 minutes

Servings: 6

Ingredients:

- 1 tablespoon avocado oil
- 32 ounces pork sausage meat
- 10 ounces canned tomatoes and jalapenos, chopped
- 10 ounces spinach
- 1 green bell pepper, chopped
- 4 cups beef stock
- 1 teaspoon onion powder
- Salt and black pepper to the taste
- 1 tablespoon cumin
- 1 tablespoon chili powder
- 1 teaspoon garlic powder
- 1 teaspoon Italian seasoning

Directions:

1. Heat up a pot with the oil over medium heat, add sausage, stir and brown for a couple of minutes on all sides.
2. Add green bell pepper, salt and pepper, stir and cook for 3 minutes.
3. Add tomatoes and jalapenos, stir and cook for 2 minutes more.
4. Add spinach, stir, cover and cook for 7 minutes.
5. Add stock, onion powder, garlic powder, chili powder, cumin, salt, pepper and Italian seasoning, stir everything, cover pot and cook for 30 minutes.
6. Uncover pot and cook soup for 15 minutes more.
7. Divide into bowls and serve.

Enjoy!

Nutrition: calories 524, fat 43, fiber 2, carbs 4, protein 26

Italian Sausage Soup

Everyone can make this amazing keto soup! It's so tasty and healthy!

Preparation time: 10 minutes

Cooking time: 30 minutes

Servings: 12

Ingredients:

- 64 ounces chicken stock
- A drizzle of avocado oil
- 1 cup heavy cream
- 10 ounces spinach
- 6 bacon slices, chopped
- 1 pound radishes, chopped
- 2 garlic cloves, minced
- Salt and black pepper to the taste
- A pinch of red pepper flakes, crushed
- 1 yellow onion, chopped
- 1 and ½ pounds hot pork sausage, chopped

Directions:

1. Heat up a pot with a drizzle of avocado oil over medium high heat, add sausage, onion and garlic, stir and brown for a few minutes.
2. Add stock, spinach and radishes, stir and bring to a simmer.
3. Add bacon, cream, salt, pepper and red pepper flakes, stir and cook for 20 minutes more.
4. Divide into bowls and serve.

Enjoy!

Nutrition: calories 291, fat 22, fiber 2, carbs 4, protein 17

Ketogenic Vegetable Recipes

Amazing Broccoli And Cauliflower Cream

This is so textured and delicious!

Preparation time: 10 minutes

Cooking time: 15 minutes

Servings: 5

Ingredients:

- 1 cauliflower head, florets separated
- 1 broccoli head, florets separated
- Salt and black pepper to the taste
- 2 garlic cloves, minced
- 2 bacon slices, chopped
- 2 tablespoons ghee

Directions:

1. Heat up a pot with the ghee over medium high heat, add garlic and bacon, stir and cook for 3 minutes.
2. Add cauliflower and broccoli florets, stir and cook for 2 minutes more.
3. Add water to cover them, cover pot and simmer for 10 minutes.
4. Add salt and pepper, stir again and blend soup using an immersion blender.

5. Simmer for a couple more minutes over medium heat, ladle into bowls and serve.

Enjoy!

Nutrition: calories 230, fat 3, fiber 3, carbs 6, protein 10

Broccoli Stew

This veggie stew is just delicious!

Preparation time: 10 minutes

Cooking time: 40 minutes

Servings: 4

Ingredients:

- 1 broccoli head, florets separated
- 2 teaspoons coriander seeds
- A drizzle of olive oil
- 1 yellow onion, chopped
- Salt and black pepper to the taste
- A pinch of red pepper, crushed
- 1 small ginger piece, chopped
- 1 garlic clove, minced
- 28 ounces canned tomatoes, pureed

Directions:

1. Put water in a pot, add salt, bring to a boil over medium high heat, add broccoli florets, steam them for 2 minutes, transfer them to a bowl filled with ice water, drain them and leave aside.

2. Heat up a pan over medium high heat, add coriander seeds, toast them for 4 minutes, transfer to a grinder, ground them and leave aside as well.

3. Heat up a pot with the oil over medium heat, add onions, salt, pepper and red pepper, stir and cook for 7 minutes.

4. Add ginger, garlic and coriander seeds, stir and cook for 3 minutes.

5. Add tomatoes, bring to a boil and simmer for 10 minutes.

6. Add broccoli, stir and cook your stew for 12 minutes.

7. Divide into bowls and serve.

Enjoy!

Nutrition: calories 150, fat 4, fiber 2, carbs 5, protein 12

Amazing Watercress Soup

A Chinese style keto soup sounds pretty amazing, doesn't it?

Preparation time: 10 minutes

Cooking time: 10 minutes

Servings: 4

Ingredients:

- 6 cup chicken stock
- ¼ cup sherry
- 2 teaspoons coconut aminos
- 6 and ½ cups watercress
- Salt and black pepper to the taste
- 2 teaspoons sesame seed
- 3 shallots, chopped
- 3 egg whites, whisked

Directions:

1. Put stock into a pot, mix with salt, pepper, sherry and coconut aminos, stir and bring to a boil over medium high heat.

2. Add shallots, watercress and egg whites, stir, bring to a boil, divide into bowls and serve with sesame seeds sprinkled on top.

Enjoy!

Nutrition: calories 50, fat 1, fiber 0, carbs 1, protein 5

Delicious Bok Choy Soup

You can even have this for dinner!

Preparation time: 10 minutes

Cooking time: 15 minutes

Servings: 4

Ingredients:

- 3 cups beef stock
- 1 yellow onion, chopped
- 1 bunch bok choy, chopped
- 1 and ½ cups mushrooms, chopped
- Salt and black pepper to the taste
- ½ tablespoon red pepper flakes
- 3 tablespoons coconut aminos
- 3 tablespoons parmesan, grated
- 2 tablespoons Worcestershire sauce
- 2 bacon strips, chopped

Directions:

1. Heat up a pot over medium high heat, add bacon, stir, cook until it until it's crispy, transfer to paper towels and drain grease.

2. Heat up the pot again over medium heat, add mushrooms and onions, stir and cook for 5 minutes.
3. Add stock, bok choy, coconut aminos, salt, pepper, pepper flakes and Worcestershire sauce, stir, cover and cook until bok choy is tender.
4. Ladle soup into bowls, sprinkle parmesan and bacon and serve.

Enjoy!

Nutrition: calories 100, fat 3, fiber 1, carbs 2, protein 6

Bok Choy Stir Fry

It's simple, it's easy and very delicious!

Preparation time: 10 minutes

Cooking time: 7 minutes

Servings: 2

Ingredients:

- 2 garlic cloves, minced
- 2 cup bok choy, chopped
- 2 bacon slices, chopped
- Salt and black pepper to the taste
- A drizzle of avocado oil

Directions:

1. Heat up a pan with the oil over medium heat, add bacon, stir and brown until it's crispy, transfer to paper towels and drain grease.

2. Return pan to medium heat, add garlic and bok choy, stir and cook for 4 minutes.
3. Add salt, pepper and return bacon, stir, cook for 1 minute more, divide between plates and serve.

Enjoy!

Nutrition: calories 50, fat 1, fiber 1, carbs 2, protein 2

Cream of Celery

This will impress you!

Preparation time: 10 minutes

Cooking time: 40 minutes

Servings: 4

Ingredients:

- 1 bunch celery, chopped
- Salt and black pepper to the taste
- 3 bay leaves
- ½ garlic head, chopped
- 2 yellow onions, chopped
- 4 cups chicken stock
- ¾ cup heavy cream
- 2 tablespoons ghee

Directions:

1. Heat up a pot with the ghee over medium high heat, add onions, salt and pepper, stir and cook for 5 minutes.
2. Add bay leaves, garlic and celery, stir and cook for 15 minutes.

3. Add stock, more salt and pepper, stir, cover pot, reduce heat and simmer for 20 minutes.
4. Add cream, stir and blend everything using an immersion blender.
5. Ladle into soup bowls and serve.

Enjoy!

Nutrition: calories 150, fat 3, fiber 1, carbs 2, protein 6

Delightful Celery Soup

It's so delightful and delicious! Try it!

Preparation time: 10 minutes

Cooking time: 25 minutes

Servings: 8

Ingredients:

- 26 ounces celery leaves and stalks, chopped
- 1 tablespoon onion flakes
- Salt and black pepper to the taste
- 3 teaspoons fenugreek powder
- 3 teaspoons veggie stock powder
- 10 ounces sour cream

Directions:

1. Put celery into a pot, add water to cover, add onion flakes, salt, pepper, stock powder and fenugreek powder, stir, bring to a boil over medium heat and simmer for 20 minutes.
2. Use an immersion blender to make your cream, add sour cream, more salt and pepper and blend again.

3. Heat up soup again over medium heat, ladle into bowls and serve.

Enjoy!

Nutrition: calories 140, fat 2, fiber 1, carbs 5, protein 10

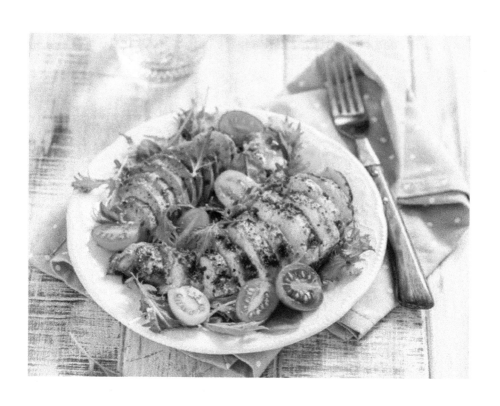

Amazing Celery Stew

This Iranian style keto stew is so tasty and easy to make!

Preparation time: 10 minutes

Cooking time: 30 minutes

Servings: 6

Ingredients:

- 1 celery bunch, roughly chopped
- 1 yellow onion, chopped
- 1 bunch green onion, chopped
- 4 garlic cloves, minced
- Salt and black pepper to the taste
- 1 parsley bunch, chopped
- 2 mint bunches, chopped
- 3 dried Persian lemons, pricked with a fork
- 2 cups water
- 2 teaspoons chicken bouillon
- 4 tablespoons olive oil

Directions:

1. Heat up a pot with the oil over medium high heat, add onion, green onions and garlic, stir and cook for 6 minutes.

2. Add celery, Persian lemons, chicken bouillon, salt, pepper and water, stir, cover pot and simmer on medium heat for 20 minutes.

3. Add parsley and mint, stir and cook for 10 minutes more.

4. Divide into bowls and serve.

Enjoy!

Nutrition: calories 170, fat 7, fiber 4, carbs 6, protein 10

Spinach Soup

It's a textured and creamy keto soup you have to try soon!

Preparation time: 10 minutes

Cooking time: 15 minutes

Servings: 8

Ingredients:

- 2 tablespoons ghee
- 20 ounces spinach, chopped
- 1 teaspoon garlic, minced
- Salt and black pepper to the taste
- 45 ounces chicken stock
- ½ teaspoon nutmeg, ground
- 2 cups heavy cream
- 1 yellow onion, chopped

Directions:

1. Heat up a pot with the ghee over medium heat, add onion, stir and cook for 4 minutes.
2. Add garlic, stir and cook for 1 minute.
3. Add spinach and stock, stir and cook for 5 minutes.

4. Blend soup with an immersion blender and heat up the soup again.
5. Add salt, pepper, nutmeg and cream, stir and cook for 5 minutes more.
6. Ladle into bowls and serve.

Enjoy!

Nutrition: calories 245, fat 24, fiber 3, carbs 4, protein 6

Delicious Mustard Greens Sauté

This is so tasty!

Preparation time: 10 minutes

Cooking time: 20 minutes

Servings: 4

Ingredients:

- 2 garlic cloves, minced
- 1 tablespoon olive oil
- 2 and ½ pounds collard greens, chopped
- 1 teaspoon lemon juice
- 1 tablespoon ghee
- Salt and black pepper to the taste

Directions:

1. Put some water in a pot, add salt and bring to a simmer over medium heat.
2. Add greens, cover and cook for 15 minutes.
3. Drain collard greens well, press out liquid and put them into a bowl.
4. Heat up a pan with the oil and the ghee over medium high heat, add collard greens, salt, pepper and garlic.

5. Stir well and cook for 5 minutes.

6. Add more salt and pepper if needed, drizzle lemon juice, stir, divide between plates and serve.

Enjoy!

Nutrition: calories 151, fat 6, fiber 3, carbs 7, protein 8

Tasty Collards Greens And Ham

This tasty dish will be ready in not time!

Preparation time: 10 minutes

Cooking time: 1 hour and 40 minutes

Servings: 4

Ingredients:

- 4 ounces ham, boneless, cooked and chopped
- 1 tablespoon olive oil
- 2 pounds collard greens, cut in medium strips
- 1 teaspoon red pepper flakes, crushed
- Salt and black pepper to the taste
- 2 cups chicken stock
- 1 yellow onion, chopped
- 4 ounces dry white wine
- 1 ounce salt pork
- ¼ cup apple cider vinegar
- ½ cup ghee, melted

Directions:

1. Heat up a pan with the oil over medium high heat, add ham and onion, stir and cook for 4 minutes.

2. Add salt pork, collard greens, stock, vinegar and wine, stir and bring to a boil.
3. Reduce heat, cover pan and cook for 1 hour and 30 minutes stirring from time to time.
4. Add ghee, discard salt pork, stir, cook everything for 10 minutes, divide between plates and serve.

Enjoy!

Nutrition: calories 150, fat 12, fiber 2, carbs 4, protein 8

Tasty Collard Greens And Tomatoes

This is just fantastic!

Preparation time: 10 minutes

Cooking time: 12 minutes

Servings:5

Ingredients:

- 1 pound collard greens
- 3 bacon strips, chopped
- ¼ cup cherry tomatoes, halved
- 1 tablespoon apple cider vinegar
- 2 tablespoons chicken stock
- Salt and black pepper to the taste

Directions:

1. Heat up a pan over medium heat, add bacon, stir and cook until it browns.

2. Add tomatoes, collard greens, vinegar, stock, salt and pepper, stir and cook for 8 minutes.
3. Add more salt and pepper, stir again gently, divide between plates and serve.

Enjoy!

Nutrition: calories 120, fat 8, fiber 1, carbs 3, protein 7

Simple Mustard Greens Dish

Everyone can make this simple keto dish! You'll see!

Preparation time: 5 minutes

Cooking time: 15 minutes

Servings: 4

Ingredients:

- 2 garlic cloves, minced
- 1 pound mustard greens, torn
- 1 tablespoon olive oil
- ½ cup yellow onion, sliced
- Salt and black pepper to the taste
- 3 tablespoons veggie stock
- ¼ teaspoon dark sesame oil

Directions:

1. Heat up a pan with the oil over medium heat, add onions, stir and brown them for 10 minutes.
2. Add garlic, stir and cook for 1 minute.
3. Add stock, greens, salt and pepper, stir and cook for 5 minutes more.

4. Add more salt and pepper and the sesame oil, toss to coat, divide between plates and serve.

Enjoy!

Nutrition: calories 120, fat 3, fiber 1, carbs 3, protein 6

Delicious Collard Greens And Poached Eggs

This will really make everyone love your cooking!

Preparation time: 10 minutes

Cooking time: 15 minutes

Servings: 6

Ingredients:

- 1 tablespoon chipotle in adobo, mashed
- 6 eggs
- 3 tablespoons ghee
- 1 yellow onion, chopped
- 2 garlic cloves, minced
- 6 bacon slices, chopped
- 3 bunches collard greens, chopped
- ½ cup chicken stock
- Salt and black pepper to the taste
- 1 tablespoon lime juice
- Some grated cheddar cheese

Directions:

1. Heat up a pan over medium high heat, add bacon, cook until it's crispy, transfer to paper towels, drain grease and leave aside.

2. Heat up the pan again over medium heat, add garlic and onion, stir and cook for 2 minutes.
3. Return bacon to the pan, stir and cook for 3 minutes more.
4. Add chipotle in adobo paste, collard greens, salt and pepper, stir and cook for 10 minutes.
5. Add stock and lime juice and stir.
6. Make 6 holes in collard greens mix, divide ghee in them, crack an egg in each hole, cover pan and cook until eggs are done.
7. Divide this between plates and serve with cheddar cheese sprinkled on top.

Enjoy!

Nutrition: calories 245, fat 20, fiber 1, carbs 5, protein 12

Collard Greens Soup

This is a keto soup even vegetarians will love!

Preparation time: 10 minutes

Cooking time: 40 minutes

Servings: 12

Ingredients:

- 1 teaspoon chili powder
- 1 tablespoon avocado oil
- 2 teaspoons smoked paprika
- 1 teaspoon cumin
- 1 yellow onion, chopped
- A pinch of red pepper flakes
- 10 cups water
- 3 celery stalks, chopped
- 3 carrots, chopped
- 15 ounces canned tomatoes, chopped
- 2 tablespoons tamari sauce
- 6 ounces canned tomato paste
- 2 tablespoons lemon juice
- Salt and black pepper to the taste

- 6 cups collard greens, stems discarded
- 1 tablespoon swerve
- 1 teaspoon garlic granules
- 1 tablespoon herb seasoning

Directions:

1. Heat up a pot with the oil over medium high heat, add cumin, pepper flakes, paprika and chili powder and stir well.
2. Add celery, onion and carrots, stir and cook for 10 minutes.
3. Add tamari sauce, tomatoes, tomato paste, water, lemon juice, salt, pepper, herb seasoning, swerve, garlic granules and collard greens, stir, bring to a boil, cover and cook for 30 minutes.
4. Stir again, ladle into bowls and serve.

Enjoy!

Nutrition: calories 150, fat 3, fiber 2, carbs 4, protein 8

Spring Green Soup

This is a fresh spring Ketogenic soup!

Preparation time: 10 minutes

Cooking time: 30 minutes

Servings: 4

Ingredients:

- 2 cups mustard greens, chopped
- 2 cups collard greens, chopped
- 3 quarts veggie stock
- 1 yellow onion, chopped
- Salt and black pepper to the taste
- 2 tablespoons coconut aminos
- 2 teaspoons ginger, grated

Directions:

1. Put the stock into a pot and bring to a simmer over medium high heat.
2. Add mustard and collard greens, onion, salt, pepper, coconut aminos and ginger, stir, cover pot and cook for 30 minutes.

3. Blend soup using an immersion blender, add more salt and pepper, heat up over medium heat, ladle into soup bowls and serve.

Enjoy!

Nutrition: calories 140, fat 2, fiber 1, carbs 3, protein 7

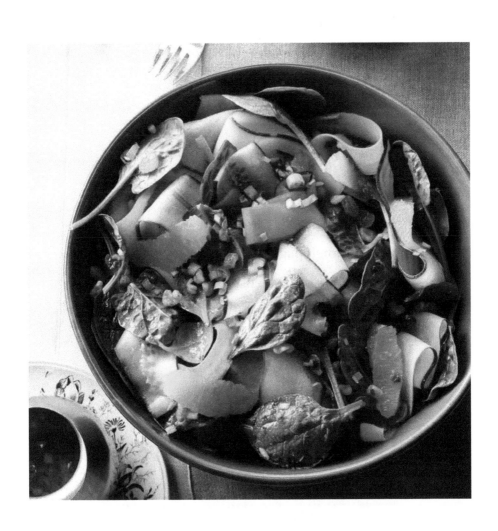

Mustard Greens And Spinach Soup

This Indian style keto soup is amazing!

Preparation time: 10 minutes

Cooking time: 15 minutes

Servings: 6

Ingredients:

- ½ teaspoon fenugreek seeds
- 1 teaspoon cumin seeds
- 1 tablespoon avocado oil
- 1 teaspoon coriander seeds
- 1 cup yellow onion, chopped
- 1 tablespoon garlic, minced
- 1 tablespoon ginger, grated
- ½ teaspoon turmeric, ground
- 5 cups mustard greens, chopped
- 3 cups coconut milk
- 1 tablespoon jalapeno, chopped
- 5 cups spinach, torn
- Salt and black pepper to the taste
- 2 teaspoons ghee

- ½ teaspoon paprika

Directions:

1. Heat up a pot with the oil over medium high heat, add coriander, fenugreek and cumin seeds, stir and brown them for 2 minutes.
2. Add onions, stir and cook for 3 minutes more.
3. Add half of the garlic, jalapenos, ginger and turmeric, stir and cook for 3 minutes more.
4. Add mustard greens and spinach, stir and sauté everything for 10 minutes.
5. Add milk, salt and pepper and blend soup using an immersion blender.
6. Heat up a pan with the ghee over medium heat, add garlic and paprika, stir well and take off heat.
7. Heat up the soup over medium heat, ladle into soup bowls, drizzle ghee and paprika all over and soup.

Enjoy!

Nutrition: calories 143, fat 6, fiber 3, carbs 7, protein 7

Roasted Asparagus

It's incredibly easy and super delicious!

Preparation time: 10 minutes

Cooking time: 10 minutes

Servings: 3

Ingredients:

- 1 asparagus bunch, trimmed
- 3 teaspoons avocado oil
- A splash of lemon juice
- Salt and black pepper to the taste
- 1 tablespoon oregano, chopped

Directions:

1. Spread asparagus spears on a lined baking sheet, season with salt and pepper, drizzle oil and lemon juice, sprinkle oregano and toss to coat well.

2. Introduce in the oven at 425 degrees F and bake for 10 minutes.

   Divide between plates and serve.

Enjoy!

Nutrition: calories 130, fat 1, fiber 1, carbs 2, protein 3

Simple Asparagus Fries

These will be ready in only 10 minutes!

Preparation time: 10 minutes

Cooking time: 10 minutes

Servings: 2

Ingredients:

- ¼ cup parmesan, grated
- 16 asparagus spears, trimmed
- 1 egg, whisked
- ½ teaspoon onion powder
- 2 ounces pork rinds

Directions:

1. Crush pork rinds and put them in a bowl.
2. Add onion powder and cheese and stir everything.
3. Roll asparagus spears in egg, then dip them in pork rind mix and arrange them all on a lined baking sheet.
4. Introduce in the oven at 425 degrees F and bake for 10 minutes.

5. Divide between plates and serve them with some sour cream on the side.

Enjoy!

Nutrition: calories 120, fat 2, fiber 2, carbs 5, protein 8

Amazing Asparagus And Browned Butter

This keto dish is very delicious and it also looks wonderful!

Preparation time: 10 minutes

Cooking time: 15 minutes

Servings: 4

Ingredients:

- 5 ounces butter
- 1 tablespoon avocado oil
- 1 and ½ pounds asparagus, trimmed
- 1 and ½ tablespoons lemon juice
- A pinch of cayenne pepper
- 8 tablespoons sour cream
- Salt and black pepper to the taste
- 3 ounces parmesan, grated
- 4 eggs

Directions:

1. Heat up a pan with 2 ounces butter over medium high heat, add eggs, some salt and pepper, stir and scramble them.

2. Transfer eggs to a blender, add parmesan, sour cream, salt, pepper and cayenne pepper and blend everything well.

3. Heat up a pan with the oil over medium high heat, add asparagus, salt and pepper, roast for a few minutes, transfer to a plate and leave them aside.

4. Heat up the pan again with the rest of the butter over medium high heat, stir until it's brown, take off heat, add lemon juice and stir well.

5. Heat up the butter again, return asparagus, toss to coat, heat up well and divide between plates.

6. Add blended eggs on top and serve.

Enjoy!

Nutrition: calories 160, fat 7, fiber 2, carbs 6, protein 10

Asparagus Frittata

It's really, really tasty!

Preparation time: 10 minutes

Cooking time: 15 minutes

Servings: 4

Ingredients:

- ¼ cup yellow onion, chopped
- A drizzle of olive oil
- 1 pound asparagus spears, cut into 1 inch pieces
- Salt and black pepper to the taste
- 4 eggs, whisked
- 1 cup cheddar cheese, grated

Directions:

1. Heat up a pan with the oil over medium high heat, add onions, stir and cook for 3 minutes.
2. Add asparagus, stir and cook for 6 minutes.
3. Add eggs, stir a bit and cook for 3 minutes.

4. Add salt, pepper and sprinkle the cheese, introduce in the oven and broil for 3 minutes.

5. Divide frittata between plates and serve.

Enjoy!

Nutrition: calories 200, fat 12, fiber 2, carbs 5, protein 14

Creamy Asparagus

It's a very creamy keto dish you can try tonight!

Preparation time: 10 minutes

Cooking time: 15 minutes

Servings: 3

Ingredients:

- 10 ounces asparagus spears, cut into medium pieces and steamed
- Salt and black pepper to the taste
- 2 tablespoons parmesan, grated
- 1/3 cup Monterey jack cheese, shredded
- 2 tablespoons mustard
- 2 ounces cream cheese
- 1/3 cup heavy cream
- 3 tablespoons bacon, cooked and crumbled

Directions:

1. Heat up a pan with the mustard, heavy cream and cream cheese over medium heat and stir well.
2. Add Monterey Jack cheese and parmesan, stir and cook until it melts.

3. Add half of the bacon and the asparagus, stir and cook for 3 minutes.
4. Add the rest of the bacon, salt and pepper, stir, cook for 5 minutes, divide between plates and serve.

Enjoy!

Nutrition: calories 256, fat 23, fiber 2, carbs 5, protein 13

Delicious Sprouts Salad

This is so fresh and full of vitamins! It's wonderful!

Preparation time: 10 minutes

Cooking time: 0 minutes

Servings: 4

Ingredients:

- 1 green apple, cored and julienned
- 1 and ½ teaspoons dark sesame oil
- 4 cups alfalfa sprouts
- Salt and black pepper to the taste
- 1 and ½ teaspoons grape seed oil
- ¼ cup coconut milk yogurt
- 4 nasturtium leaves

Directions:

1. In a salad bowl mix sprouts with apple and nasturtium.
2. Add salt, pepper, sesame oil, grape seed oil and coconut yogurt, toss to coat and divide between plates.
3. Serve right away.

Enjoy!

Nutrition: calories 100, fat 3, fiber 1, carbs 2, protein 6

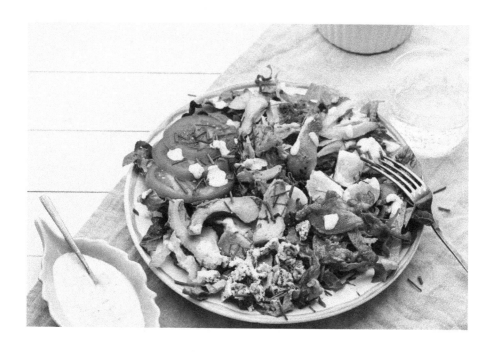

Roasted Radishes

If you don't have time to cook a complex dinner tonight, then try this recipe!

Preparation time: 10 minutes

Cooking time: 35 minutes

Servings: 2

Ingredients:

- 2 cups radishes, cut in quarters
- Salt and black pepper to the taste
- 2 tablespoons ghee, melted
- 1 tablespoon chives, chopped
- 1 tablespoon lemon zest

Directions:

1. Spread radishes on a lined baking sheet.
2. Add salt and pepper, chives, lemon zest and ghee, toss to coat and bake in the oven at 375 degrees F for 35 minutes.
3. Divide between plates and serve.

Enjoy!

Nutrition: calories 122, fat 12, fiber 1, carbs 3, protein 14

Radish Hash Browns

Do you want to learn how to make this tasty keto dish? Then, pay attention.

Preparation time: 10 minutes

Cooking time: 10 minutes

Servings: 4

Ingredients:

- ½ teaspoon onion powder
- 1 pound radishes, shredded
- ½ teaspoon garlic powder
- Salt and black pepper to the taste
- 4 eggs
- 1/3 cup parmesan, grated

Directions:

1. In a bowl, mix radishes with salt, pepper, onion and garlic powder, eggs and parmesan and stir well.
2. Spread this on a lined baking sheet, introduce in the oven at 375 degrees F and bake for 10 minutes.
3. Divide hash browns between plates and serve.

Enjoy!

Nutrition: calories 80, fat 5, fiber 2, carbs 5, protein 7

Crispy Radishes

It's a great keto idea!

Preparation time: 10 minutes

Cooking time: 20 minutes

Servings: 4

Ingredients:

- Cooking spray
- 15 radishes, sliced
- Salt and black pepper to the taste
- 1 tablespoon chives, chopped

Directions:

1. Arrange radish slices on a lined baking sheet and spray them with cooking oil.

2. Season with salt and pepper and sprinkle chives, introduce in the oven at 375 degrees F and bake for 10 minutes.
3. Flip them and bake for 10 minutes more.
4. Serve them cold.

Enjoy!

Nutrition: calories 30, fat 1, fiber 0.4, carbs 1, protein 0.1

Creamy Radishes

It's a creamy and tasty keto veggie dish!

Preparation time: 10 minutes

Cooking time: 25 minutes

Servings: 1

Ingredients:

- 7 ounces radishes, cut in halves
- 2 tablespoons sour cream
- 2 bacon slices
- 1 tablespoon green onion, chopped
- 1 tablespoon cheddar cheese, grated
- Hot sauce to the taste
- Salt and black pepper to the taste

Directions:

1. Put radishes into a pot, add water to cover, bring to a boil over medium heat, cook them for 10 minutes and drain.
2. Heat up a pan over medium high heat, add bacon, cook until it's crispy, transfer to paper towels, drain grease, crumble and leave aside.

3. Return pan to medium heat, add radishes, stir and sauté them for 7 minutes.
4. Add onion, salt, pepper, hot sauce and sour cream, stir and cook for 7 minutes more.
5. Transfer to a plate, top with crumbled bacon and cheddar cheese and serve.

Enjoy!

Nutrition: calories 340, fat 23, fiber 3, carbs 6, protein 15

Radish Soup

Oh my God! This tastes divine!

Preparation time: 10 minutes

Cooking time: 20 minutes

Servings: 4

Ingredients:

- 2 bunches radishes, cut in quarters
- Salt and black pepper to the taste
- 6 cups chicken stock
- 2 stalks celery, chopped
- 3 tablespoons coconut oil
- 6 garlic cloves, minced
- 1 yellow onion, chopped

Directions:

1. Heat up a pot with the oil over medium heat, add onion, celery and garlic, stir and cook for 5 minutes.
2. Add radishes, stock, salt and pepper, stir, bring to a boil, cover and simmer for 15 minutes.
3. Divide into soup bowls and serve.

Enjoy!

Nutrition: calories 120, fat 2, fiber 1, carbs 3, protein 10

Tasty Avocado Salad

This is very tasty and refreshing!

Preparation time: 10 minutes

Cooking time: 0 minutes

Servings: 4

Ingredients:

- 2 avocados, pitted and mashed
- Salt and black pepper to the taste
- ¼ teaspoon lemon stevia
- 1 tablespoon white vinegar
- 14 ounces coleslaw mix
- Juice from 2 limes
- ¼ cup red onion, chopped
- ¼ cup cilantro, chopped
- 2 tablespoons olive oil

Directions:

1. Put coleslaw mix in a salad bowl.

   Add avocado mash and onions and toss to coat.

2. In a bowl, mix lime juice with salt, pepper, oil, vinegar and stevia and stir well.

3. Add this to salad, toss to coat, sprinkle cilantro and serve.

Enjoy!

Nutrition: calories 100, fat 10, fiber 2, carbs 5, protein 8

Avocado And Egg Salad

You will make it again for sure!

Preparation time: 10 minutes

Cooking time: 7 minutes

Servings: 4

Ingredients:

- 4 cups mixed lettuce leaves, torn
- 4 eggs
- 1 avocado, pitted and sliced
- ¼ cup mayonnaise
- 2 teaspoons mustard
- 2 garlic cloves, minced
- 1 tablespoon chives, chopped
- Salt and black pepper to the taste

Directions:

1. Put water in a pot, add some salt, add eggs, bring to a boil over medium high heat, boil for 7 minutes, drain, cool, peel and chop them.
2. In a salad bowl, mix lettuce with eggs and avocado.

3. Add chives and garlic, some salt and pepper and toss to coat.
4. In a bowl, mix mustard with mayo, salt and pepper and stir well.
5. Add this to salad, toss well and serve right away.

Enjoy!

Nutrition: calories 234, fat 12, fiber 4, carbs 7, protein 12

Avocado And Cucumber Salad

You will ask for more! It's such a tasty summer salad!

Preparation time: 10 minutes

Cooking time: 0 minutes

Servings: 4

Ingredients:

- 1 small red onion, sliced
- 1 cucumber, sliced
- 2 avocados, pitted, peeled and chopped
- 1 pound cherry tomatoes, halved
- 2 tablespoons olive oil
- ¼ cup cilantro, chopped
- 2 tablespoons lemon juice
- Salt and black pepper to the taste

Directions:

1. In a large salad bowl, mix tomatoes with cucumber, onion and avocado and stir.
2. Add oil, salt, pepper and lemon juice and toss to coat well.
3. Serve cold with cilantro on top.

Enjoy!

Nutrition: calories 140, fat 4, fiber 2, carbs 4, protein 5

Delicious Avocado Soup

You will adore this special and delicious keto soup!

Preparation time: 10 minutes

Cooking time: 10 minutes

Servings: 4

Ingredients:

- 2 avocados, pitted, peeled and chopped
- 3 cups chicken stock
- 2 scallions, chopped
- Salt and black pepper to the taste
- 2 tablespoons ghee
- 2/3 cup heavy cream

Directions:

1. Heat up a pot with the ghee over medium heat, add scallions, stir and cook for 2 minutes.
2. Add 2 and ½ cups stock, stir and simmer for 3 minutes.

3. In your blender, mix avocados with the rest of the stock, salt, pepper and heavy cream and pulse well.
4. Add this to the pot, stir well, cook for 2 minutes and season with more salt and pepper.
5. Stir well, ladle into soup bowls and serve.

Enjoy!

Nutrition: calories 332, fat 23, fiber 4, carbs 6, protein 6

Delicious Avocado And Bacon Soup

Have you ever heard about such a delicious keto soup? Then it's time you find out more about it!

Preparation time: 10 minutes

Cooking time: 10 minutes

Servings: 4

Ingredients:

- 2 avocados, pitted and cut in halves
- 4 cups chicken stock
- 1/3 cup cilantro, chopped
- Juice of ½ lime
- 1 teaspoon garlic powder
- ½ pound bacon, cooked and chopped
- Salt and black pepper to the taste

Directions:

1. Put stock in a pot and bring to a boil over medium high heat.
2. In your blender, mix avocados with garlic powder, cilantro, lime juice, salt and pepper and blend well.

3. Add this to stock and blend using an immersion blender.
4. Add bacon, more salt and pepper the taste, stir, cook for 3 minutes, ladle into soup bowls and serve.

Enjoy!

Nutrition: calories 300, fat 23, fiber 5, carbs 6, protein 17

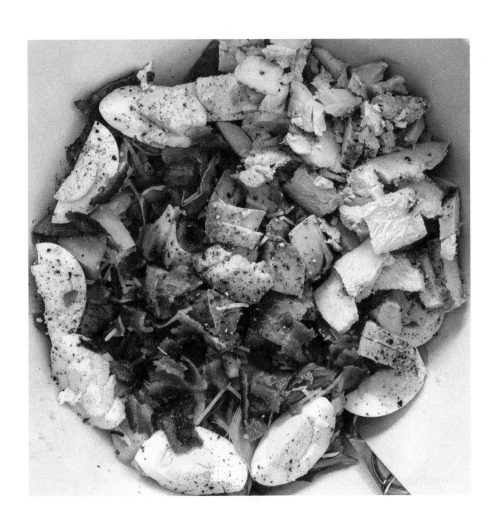

Thai Avocado Soup

This is a great and exotic soup!

Preparation time: 10 minutes

Cooking time: 10 minutes

Servings: 4

Ingredients:

- 1 cup coconut milk
- 2 teaspoons Thai green curry paste
- 1 avocado, pitted, peeled and chopped
- 1 tablespoon cilantro, chopped
- Salt and black pepper to the taste
- 2 cups veggie stock
- Lime wedges for serving

Directions:

1. In your blender, mix avocado with salt, pepper, curry paste and coconut milk and pulse well.
2. Transfer this to a pot and heat up over medium heat.
3. Add stock, stir, bring to a simmer and cook for 5 minutes.

4. Add cilantro, more salt and pepper, stir, cook for 1 minute more, ladle into soup bowls and serve with lime wedges on the side.

Enjoy!

Nutrition: calories 240, fat 4, fiber 2, carbs 6, protein 12

Conclusion

This is really a life changing cookbook. It shows you everything you need to know about the Ketogenic diet and it helps you get started.

You now know some of the best and most popular Ketogenic recipes in the world.

We have something for everyone's taste!

So, don't hesitate too much and start your new life as a follower of the Ketogenic diet!

Get your hands on this special recipes collection and start cooking in this new, exciting and healthy way!

Have a lot of fun and enjoy your Ketogenic diet!